MW01535016

Introduction TO
IRIDOLOGY

by Dr. Donald R. Bamer

WOODLAND PUBLISHING
Pleasant Grove, UT

© 1996
Woodland Publishing, Inc.
P.O. Box 160
Pleasant Grove, UT
84062

The information in this book is for educational purposes only iand is not recommended as a means of diagnosing or treating an illness. All matters concerning physical and mental health should be supervised by a health practitioner knowledgeable in treating that particular condition. Neither the publisher nor author directly or indirectly dispense medical advice, nor do they prescribe any remedies or assume any responsibility for those who choose to treat themselves.

Table of Contents

Section 1

WHAT IS IRIDOLOGY?

Iridology is the study and practice that uses the eye, more specifically the iris, to detect changes, abnormalities and disorders within the body, as well the severity of such. The iris can reveal the constitution and inherent weaknesses in all areas of one's body, as well as the level of health or homeostasis of these areas.

Iridology involves analyzing the structures of the iris, the portion of the eye that carries the color. The iris is made up of thousands of fibers, the which are the main indicators used in iridology study. It is the fibers correspond to various regions and organs of the body, and that indicate the level of health and/or types of disorder that area is experiencing.

The Eyes are the Windows to the Body

The scriptures have always told us that the "eye is the window to the soul" and we know that it is also very reflective of the a person's mood. We can tell if they are apathetic, sad, or just don't feel well. There are many, many things we can tell about how a person feels just by looking at their eyes.

One hundred and fifty years ago, German doctors began to realize that the eye also served as a diagnostic tool, something that would note changes or problems in tissues in certain areas of the body. The original emphasis was on the back of the eye, the portion called the retina. The retina is diagnostic—we can see indications there of many possible ailments or disorders, like *Diabetes mellitus* (sugar diabetes), brain tumors, blocking of the arteries and so forth. Many things can be seen in the retina, but doctors realized that although the retina told some things about the body (more than they knew before), the retina also had its shortcomings because the information it provided was limited. This led them to continue their search. As the researchers analyzed the eye, more and more they began to appreciate and see the patterns and the correlation between the blood vessels which were occurring on the sclera (the white of the eye) and what was occurring on the back and the iris of the eye. In fact, as their research continued they even found the iris (the colored part) had specific patterns and changes that told them still more about what changes and or problems a person could be experiencing. As they went further and further they realized that the whole eye represented the whole body and that the true way to analyze a person holistically was through the analysis of the whole eye and its relationship to the body.

WHAT THE EYES SHOW

Through the various patterns and colors that appear in the iris, it is possible to detect underactive organs or tissues and overactive organs and tissues. The eyes show the problem regardless of what stage it is in, even from its presymptomatic phase. Like a cavity in a tooth, it is detectable very early, but if allowed to progress, can create quite a problem.

The human body is a highly sophisticated piece of machinery, far superior to any computer or machine. We are extremely "computerized" with many remote test and treatment points. Our feet, hands, ears and eyes serve as diagnostic sensors and excellent body treatment outlets. To treat the body through the feet we use foot reflexology; likewise, to treat the body through the hand we use hand reflexology; and finally, to treat the body through the ear we use ear reflexology/auriculotherapy. Although the body can be treated through the eyes, the eyes are normally reserved for biological analysis. The body runs using electric currents and each organ and tissue has a specific vibration—normal, underactive, overactive and degenerative. The fibers of the iris are sensitive to the changing vibrations of these tissues and organs. Although iridology and sclerology may seem somewhat magical, their procedures are based upon solid principles. It is not usually necessary to cut, poke and draw blood to understand what is causing a person's problems, which has been commonly done in most Western cultures. The Chinese functioned quite well for over 2,000 years without ever dissecting or invading the body in any way to analyze a health problem. In fact, their belief was that one could only truly understand a person's problems by evaluating them while they were "intact" and in their own environment.

There are over ninety different organs and tissues represented in the eye. The eye patterns are so specific for each individual they are believed to be far more accurate and permanent than even fingerprints. Iridology, like many things that have been used successfully for hundreds of years, is just now being understood. Not because it has changed, but because we have changed—changed in our open-mindedness enough to accept something that works even if we can't completely understand it. Our understanding of the energy systems, meridians and nervous system has opened our eyes to the complexity of the human body. Although iridology as a science has only been in this country fifty to sixty years, its accuracy and simplicity of use has accelerated it to the forefront of natural alternative health analysis. Reflex testing, including muscle response testing, cannot reveal the depth of a problem, its cause, or even what else may be involved. Only the complete eye-body analysis can give this information. Muscle reflex testing in conjunction with the iris analysis is beneficial in selecting herbal or other natural products.

SUMMARY OF IRIDOLOGY BENEFITS

The following summarize some of the many possible benefits of using iridology and/or sclerology treatments:

1. Show weak areas
2. Reveal inflammation, acute and chronic
3. Reveal degeneration
4. Show healing—help evaluate a health program
5. Show hidden causes to symptoms
6. Show interrelationship between body functions
7. Show the brain and higher thought centers
8. Used for prevention—stop the illness before it starts
9. Show food allergies
10. Show diverticuli/bowel pockets
11. Show ph imbalance
12. Show arthritic signs
13. Show heredity tendencies
14. Show diabetic patterns

15. Show vitamin/mineral deficiencies
16. Show possible yeast overgrowth
17. Show possible parasitic infection

Iris Color

The color of a person's eyes depends mainly upon his or her genetic configuration. There are several theories about color and the number of basic colors. Some say there are but two basic colors—blue and brown—while others feel that hazel (a combination of both) should be included.

For the purpose of our studies it is more important to concern ourselves with the layers which are pigmented and iris color changes rather than the number of basic colors. As will be seen later, it is not uncommon for a patient that appears to have brown eyes change eye color while undergoing treatment.

Special Iridology Terminology

The following gives commonly used terms and phrases and how they possibly may be used.

1) The term *collarette* corresponds to the autonomic nerve wreath.
2) The term *sphincter pupillae* corresponds to the stomach ring.
3) The term *Fuchs crypts* corresponds to closed lesions.
4) The term *contraction furrows* corresponds to nerve rings/ psychological stress rings/ psychosomatic stress rings.
5) The term *neurasthenic ring* is the pupillary pigment border.
6) The terms *freckle* or *psoric spots* are called pigmented nervi/drug spots/ mineral deposits/pathological polychromia.
7) The term *Wolffian bodies* correspond to the lymphatic tophi/psoric spots/sectoral hetechromia.

Historical Background of Iridology

It has been said that the eyes are the window to the soul, but within the last 150 years it has been realized that the eyes are also the window to the body. Indian medicine men have been known to sit and study the eyes of their patients for long periods of time before prescribing herbs or other remedies for their ailments. Shepherds would study the eyes of their sheep to tell when these animals were beginning to develop potential problems and need various remedies. One particular sign they looked for is an iris sign we call "radii solaris." The Cauldeans are known to have studied and recorded changes in the irises of their friends and relatives as long ago as 3000 years, believing these changes to have an astronomical cause and significance.

Hippocrates was probably the first to realize that there was a definite link between signs in the eyes and changes in the body. He concentrated his efforts on the posterior aspect of the eye and established the beginning of what we use today as a basic ophthalmic exam.

Analysis of the posterior eye remained the significant area of examination up to the mid-1800s. This began to change when a boy named Ignatz Peczely noticed that when an owl he was playing with became injured, a mark suddenly appeared in the iris of the owl's eye and on the same side of the injury. Thus was the discovery of a phenomenon we now call *Opthalmic-Somatic Analysis* (Iridology).

Although completely unaware of the phenomenon he was observing, he remained very curious of his findings. This led him into medical school and eventually into a hospital in Budapest, where he furthered his knowledge in this new phenomenon. Here he was able to observe and examine all patients as they were admitted and discharged. Upon their admission, Dr. Peczely would study their case histories, then he would examine very carefully their irises, taking great efforts to draw, in color, a picture of their irises in exact detail. He would again draw a picture of their irises as they were released. He noticed that a pattern was developing and it was very consistent. As an example, when a person had a liver condition it always showed at eight o'clock in the right iris. As they condition as treated, the sign would either change or disappear. He was constantly being exposed to a large variety of patients and complaints, thus enabling him to begin forming a basic chart/map of the iris that corresponded to the location of organs and tissues.

While continuing to improve and update the chart, he wrote the first book on iridology, *Discovery in the Realm of Nature and the Art of Healing.* His book so excited the medical profession in Germany that they began writing about him and his discovery.

Some of the other great people in the historical development of iridology were: Dr. Nils Liliquist, a Swedish homeopath who worked with toxic appearances in the iris from vaccinations and was first to bring iridology to America in the early 1900s; Dr. J. Haskell Kritzer, M.D., who wrote a text book, *Iris Diagnosis and Guide in Treatment;* Dr. Henry Lindlar, M.D., Chicago; and Dr. Henry Lahn, M.D., Austria. Each added significantly to the research and development of this phenomenon.

For many years what was taught in this country was the information that was originally brought over by Dr. Liliquist and later updated, at least to that point in time, by Dr. Lahn and Dr. Lindlar. However, in Germany, a more in-depth research program had begun and is still in progress today. This research began to discover the significance of the whole eye, not just the iris. That research included the retina, sclera and scleral vessels, iris, palpabrae, and even the caruncle, for each of these structures is unique. The main significance is their correlative ability, giving more than just one sign for a problem. Because of the use of the whole eye, the Germans have renamed this science *Opthalmic-Somatic Analysis,* instead of iris analysis.

Ophthalmic-Somatic Analysis now became the key diagnostic science and as late as 1979 new research material was made available from which the most up-to-date iridology chart now available has been produced.

So we see that the eye is very valuable for us to use as a diagnostic tool for most disorders that plague humankind. But just being able to identify a problem area is not enough. We must also know how to treat the patient's condition holistically, using various therapies for treatment and to monitor the healing through the eye. The following gives a detailed outline of iridology, its benefits, and its main components of study.

I.   Functions of Iridology
    A.   Iridology shows major and minor areas
       1. Inflammation
          a. Chronic
          b. Acute
       2. Poor elimination
       3. Acidity/Alkalinity
       4. Hypo-functioning organs
       5. Hyper-functioning organs
       6. Areas of ischemia
       7. Areas of anemia
       8. Underlying causes of symptoms
       9. Inherent weaknesses
       10. Acquired weaknesses

11. Diverticulitis
12. Vitamin and mineral deficiencies
13. Poor assimilation

II. Anatomy and Neurology of the Eye Motor
  A. Oculomoter, inferior and superior
    1. Superior branch
    2. Inferior branch
  B. Trochlear IV Cranial Nerve
  C. Abducens VI Cranial Nerve
  D. Autonomic nervous system
  E. Sympathetic innervation comes via the superior cervical ganglion.
  F. Parasympathetic innervation comes via the the cranial nerve (Edinger-Westphal nucleus and ciliary ganglion).
  G. Both the sphincter and dilater muscles have a sympathetic and parasympathetic innervation.

III. Blood Supply
  A. Opthalmic Artery
    1.Origin: from internal carotid artery at the end of cavernous sinus
    2.Branches:
      a. In orbit to surrounding parts
      b. In orbit to eyeball
  B. Central Artery
    1. Eyeball
    2. Macula
  C. Venous drainage of eyeball
    1. Retina drained by veins that accompany branches and trunk of central arteries.
    2.Outer coats drained by vorticose veins in outer layer of choroid. These converge and drain into the superior ophthalmic vein.

IV. Accessory Items of the Anterior Eye
   A. *Sclera:* The sclera/white of the eye is significant for two
   reasons: (1) It is an area where much plaquing occurs,
   both yellow and white. These are secondary indications of
   lipid/cholesterol metabolic problems within the body. It
   often points to a liver dysfunction. (2) Scleral vessels are
   very significant as indicators pointing to a problem area in
   the body. There are vessels which indicate a back-pressure
   in the vascular system such as would be found with hem-
   orrhoids.
   B. *Palpabrae:* The inferior palpabrae/ eyelid often shows
   pigmentation changes such as liver spots when there is a
   liver dysfunction. This is a good confirmation test. The
   palpabrae, because of its rich blood supply, is an excellent
   area to detect systemic anemia. Under these conditions the
   palpabrae appears very white and bleached out.
   C. *Pupillary response:* The pupil is formed by two muscles,
   dilator pupillae and sphincter pupillae. The expansion and
   contraction of the pupil is an excellent way to evaluate the
   sphincter control throughout the whole body. The pupil is
   also a very good indicator of adrenal dysfunction. A wide
   pupil indicates adrenal weakness and possible exhaustion.
   A very tight pupil indicates hyper-adrenalism, thus overactivity. This is a very significant sign because the adrenals
   are the glands of stress and play a major role in common
   pathological conditions of today such as hypoglycemia and
   diabetes mellitus.
   D. *Caruncle:* The caruncle, the little fatty ball nasal-ward
   in the corner of the eye, tends to attract much triglyceride
   and cholesterol plaquing and will begin showing signs
   often long before any other part of the anterior eye.

Illustration A

IRIDOLOGY CHART

Donald R. Bamer B.S.D.C.

Published by the National Iridology Association, Tulsa, Oklahoma. All rights reserved.

Iris Layers

The iris is composed of four separate layers, but only three are considered significant. They are, from anterior to posterior:

1. Anterior Border Layer (actually two layers)
   This layer is a modification of the middle stromal layer of the iris. It is composed of two layers: an anterior fibroblastic layer and a posterior pigmented layer. This posterior pigmented layer is the layer that has a great deal to do with the actual iris color.

2. Stromal Layer

3. Posterior Epithelium Layer
   It is the posterior ephithelium layer that is heavily pigmented with black and brown granules.

Section 2

HOW IRIDOLOGY WORKS

While in the maternal uterus, ophthalmic development begins from the frontal lobe of the brain. The eye, especially the iris, has a rich supply of neuro-ectodermal tissue. The iris has been estimated to contain over 28,000 individual nerve fibers mingled with stromal fibers. (This combination is extremely sensitive to nerve impulses from the automatic nervous system.) Since the brain is the ultimate control of the body, it must know the complete condition of all organs and tissues of the body at all times. This is accomplished by constant flow of both afferent and efferent impulses to and from all parts of the body.

Certain neuron cells (or aggregate of cells) in the brain respond continuously to these impulses from the areas they control. These impulses are carried via the autonomic nervous system, both sympathetic and parasympathetic. This system feeds directly into the iris via the Edinger-Westphal nucleus (parasympathetic) and via the sympathetic ganglion in the upper thoracic spine. Since the iris has such a rich supply of highly sensitive neuro-ectodermal fibers, the iris functions like a remote television picture tube, giving us a complete neurological picture of the body at all times by the reflex of neurological impulses. The significance of these impulses to the examiner is that they are at a frequency that corresponds to their health condition or any one of four stages of inflammation: acute, subacute, chronic, and degenerative.

INTERPRETING IRIS SIGNS

The interpretation of iris signs is done by noting two things:
1. A pigmentation change
2. A pattern change

The pigmentation changes correspond to stages of inflammation; the following outline the different inflammation stages:
1. Acute—white
2. Subacute—light gray
3. Chronic—dark gray
4. Degenerative/Destructive—black

Acute inflammation (white) in that area indicates that there is increased activity in the area of the body that corresponds to that particular section of the eye, which would be expected in any increased inflammation state, some of these being increased temperature, increased nerve function, and edema. These changes in this area cause the frequency of the nerve impulses going to the brain to be much higher than they would normally be. This change in frequency is being felt at the same time in the iris fibers. These fibers will also vibrate at a higher frequency, which makes the area that they represent appear much whiter than adjacent areas.

A subacute (light gray) condition is very similar to acute but of a lesser degree. This iris fiber frequency is still elevated but not to the degree that it was in the acute condition. Thus, the color will appear to be more gray than white.

A chronic (dark gray) condition requires our special attention for it is the underlying cause in most cases. In most cases, when a person has an acute condition the body is responding and the patient is aware of the condition and the area of disturbance. But in the chronic state, these are the areas that the patient has either learned to live with or is operating at a subclinical level, as often is the case when the symptoms have been continuously suppressed through drug therapy. The area now is no longer performing its functions adequately, thus the whole body is forced to relieve some of the burden.

An example would be a chronic lung condition. Here the patient probably has no continuous problems, but more likely is very susceptible to bronchitis, pneumonia, etc. Yet this weakened pneumonic tissue now is no longer performing to its maximum abilities, one being oxygen/carbon dioxide exchange. Lack of adequate uptake of oxygen can lead to generalized hypoxia throughout the body. Also, more importantly, the lack of the lungs' ability to discharge carbon dioxide causes it to be changed in the body to carbonic acid, thus placing an additional burden on the kidneys.

A destructive/degenerative (black) condition is the most serious sign that can be found in the iris. It indicates there is or has been destruction of the actual organ in that area, thus indicating a highly cancerous or precancerous condition. These should alert the examiner to request further lab work of a cancer screening nature immediately. These organs are placing a tremendous burden on the body because of their dysfunction.

These stages of inflammation correlate directly with the

activity of the various organs of the body. When an organ is in an acute inflammatory state, it is also overactive to that same degree and by the same token, underactive by the degree of chronicity indicated. Thereby these color changes allow us not only the ability to evaluate stages of inflammation, but also to determine functional changes within the organs themselves.

Somatic Constitution (Pattern Changes)

Since the fibers of the iris represent the structural soundness of any given area, we can use this to tell us the structural strength of any given area. We can evaluate it for possible inherent weaknesses, defect signs or other structural problems, or just as important, lack of problems. Somatic constitution is set up in three categories:

1. GOOD. A good constitution is where the lines are straight and reasonably close together. This represents the body of someone with high recuperative capabilities. Once a person begins to receive the proper care, he or she will bounce back very fast. There are virtually no significant weaknesses visible.
2. FAIR. This person's iris fibers are not as close and tend to be fairly wavy. There is usually evidence of several lacuna (pockets). Like the person with the good constitution, this person tends to do fairly well when receiving the proper care, even though he or she has some inherent weaknesses.
3. POOR. The person with this type of constitution must work continuously to keep the body free from disease. The fibers are widespread and there is multiple lacuna or crypts (pockets) in the iris, indicating inherent weaknesses in these areas. These people also tend to be of the psychologi-

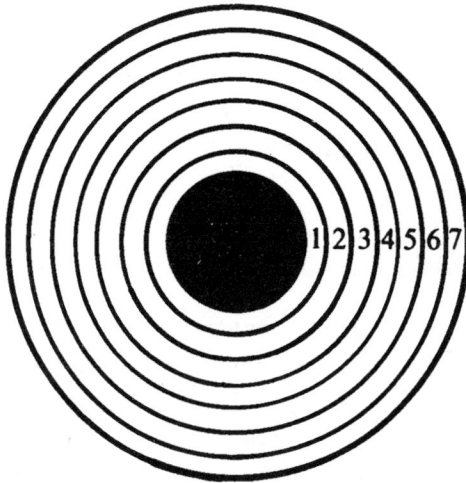

Illustration B: The iris zones

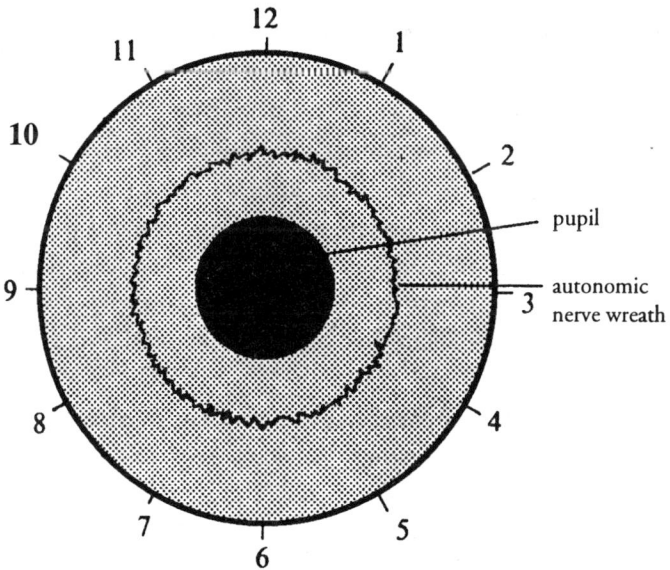

Illustration C: This iris is laid out neurologically like a clock

cal nature that they lack persistence and tend to give in easily. Often this type of person does not want to put forth any effort for good health or even accept the responsibility for it. This person will respond, but usually not 100 percent, and has to work very hard to attain a high level of recuperation.

FINDING THE ZONES

The iris develops neurologically from the pupil outward. There are a total of seven concentric zones. Each zone corresponds to certain organs and tissues and acts as a rough guide in understanding the iris. The following gives each zone and their corresponding body areas and organs.

ZONE 1 Gastric mucosa

ZONE 2 Complete intestinal tract, both small and large

ZONE 3 Heart, pancreas, pituitary gland, adrenal glands, aorta, gall bladder, solar plexis, parathyroid, uterus/ prostate pineal

ZONE 4 Bronchial tubes

ZONE 5 Brain and reproductive organs

ZONE 6 Spleen, thyroid, liver, kidneys and spine

ZONE 7 This zone is lineated into a superior and inferior section. The inferior contains lymphatic and circulatory systems, motor and sensory nerves. The superior aspect reflects changes in the sweat glands and skin.

See Illustration B for a more complete representation of the iris/body zone concept.

Section 3

ORGAN SIGNS

In addition to the irregular fibers and/or color changes in an area, research has identified several specific signs that are indications of inherited weaknesses. It was once thought in this country that there were both inherited and acquired weaknesses, but research involving thousands of people, especially families, shows that all of the signs in the iris are inherited. Thus, all inherited signs usually appear by the age of six.

What we have found to be acquired is not a weakness of any particular area because we are what our parents are, at least physically. What we actually acquire is the health condition of that area and all areas of our bodies. The color in an area reflects how we have treated our bodies or an area of dysfunction—that is what we have developed. That is something we have control over and even though we cannot change a structural weakness that has formed, based upon its genetic blueprint, we can alter the color/health state of that or any other area of our body. Unless there has been an injury that has altered our structures, these structures should not be expected to disappear. Refer to the following for a comprehensive list of organ signs.

LEAF LACUNA: This is commonly seen in the thoracic region of the iris, and is common to lung or heart weakness.

OPEN LACUNA: This is a very common sign and is seen anywhere. Compared to the leaf lacuna, the open lacuna indicates an area that is weaker.

CRYPT: Although it can be seen anywhere, it is normally seen in the glandular zone. When several are seen and they are dark, this is an indication of glandular problems such as *Diabetes mellitus,* hypoglycemia, etc.

OPEN CRYPT: Like the open lacuna it can be seen anywhere and has the same comparative value to the crypt as did the open lacuna to the leaf lacuna.

KIDNEY MEDUSA: Inherited kidney weakness will usually show with this sign. This sign, like the others, can be seen anywhere in the iris and wherever seen indicates an inherited weakness, but it is usually seen in the kidney zone.

LIVER STAKE: This is the sign most often seen in the liver zone when there is an inherited weakness present. The base of the triangle is on the outer edge of the iris and the tip points towards the pupil.

DEFECT SIGNS: This sign is not made of the combination of these: dot, spearhead, and comma or fish hook, but only one will be seen in any particular area. They are normally seen very near an inherited weakness. They are tar black in color and signify an area that is more than just weak, but in fact an area, that if allowed to become chronic, is susceptible to becoming cancerous much faster than adjacent areas. Thus the name *defect* requires much more attention than just a weakened area.

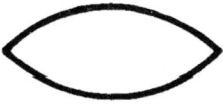

LEAF LACUNA

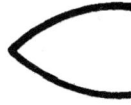

OPEN LACUNA

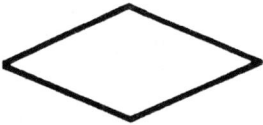

CRYPT

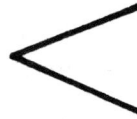

OPEN CRYPT

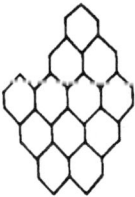

HONEY COMB

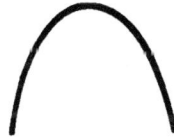

KIDNEY MEDUSSA

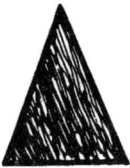

LIVER STAKE

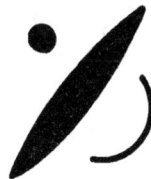

DEFECT SIGN

Illustration D: The Organ Signs

HONEYCOMB: This sign has very significant meanings. It is not an inherited weakness, but an indication of a functional problem of metabolism occurring at that location. This sign has possibilities of diminishing as the problem is corrected.

PUPILLARY CHANGES

The pupil is an opening in the eye that sits medial-nasalward in the eye. These impressions exit the optic nerve and from this we have vision. The pupil also contracts to close out light and to focus on close objects. This contraction is accomplished by the action of a muscle surrounding the pupil named *sphincter pupillae*. The pupil expands to allow more light in and to focus on objects further away. This expansion/dilation of the pupil is accomplished by the dilator pupillae.

Both of these muscles are under direct control of the autonomic nervous system, parasympathetic, and sympathetic. Whenever there is pressure on the nerve root such as in the case with a spinal subluxation, the pupil will flatten across from the area serviced by that nerve supply. An example of this would be if there were nerve root pressure in the upper thoracic spine, the pupil would flatten on the side of the greatest interference and across from the lungs and upper respiratory region, all noted on the Iridology Chart, Illustration A. Thus, the pupil tells us where there is nerve interference and which areas it is affecting.

The lining of the pupil has been found to be very helpful in detecting metabolic and pathological problems. It has been noted that the pupillary lining can become very irregular when the patient is having a glucose tolerance problem, especially *Diabetes mellitus*. A urinalysis and glucose screening test should be accomplished on all of these patients.

Section 4

IRIS SIGNS

The following explanations give an introductory list of the most common iris signs, as well as their general indications and herbal treatments. The iris signs are very helpful in determining the area of the body that is suffering, the severity of the disorder, and sometimes the length the problem has existed.

For a more complete and in-depth description of the signs and their treatments, refer to this booklet's companion publication, *Practical Iridology and Sclerology*, also by Dr. Donald Bamer.

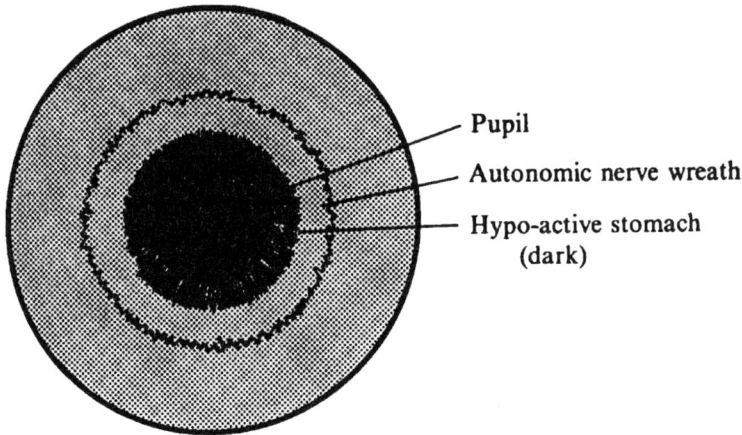

Pupil

Autonomic nerve wreath

Hypo-active stomach
(dark)

Stomach (Hypoactive)

A hypoactive/underactive stomach is probably one of the most subtle causes of malnutrition known to man. When this condition exists, there is a dark ring around the pupil in the stomach zone of the iris. This ring is called the "stomach ring. If the ring is white, the dysfunction is one of overactivity; if dark, the dysfunction is one of underactivity.

Some common symptoms of a hypoactive stomach include easy nausea, frequent belching and burping after meals, stomach and bowel gas, and a general feeling of weakness. These people are suffering from malnutrition because their foods are not being broken down adequately and thus not absorbed.

TREATMENT CONSIDERATIONS

A combination of papaya mint is very effective in combatting indigestion. An enzyme combination containing Betaine HCl, salt, bromelain, lipaise, mycozyme, pancreatin, papain and pepsin may also be helpful. Safflower is also a natural nutritional aid for the digestive system.

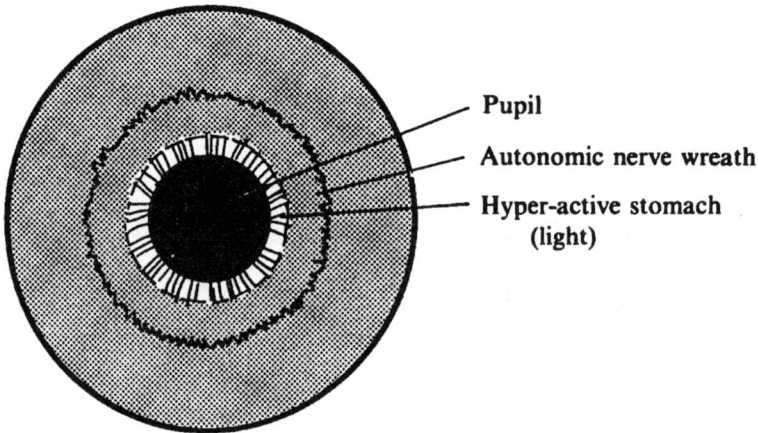

Pupil
Autonomic nerve wreath
Hyper-active stomach (light)

Stomach (Hyperactive)

When the stomach is hyperactive, whether acidic or alkaline, it will show as a white ring around the pupil. This ring has been named, and rightfully so, a "stomach ring." Some of the symptoms that can be associated with this sign are heartburn and sensitivity to such items as coffee, tea, alcohol, tobacco, citrus fruits, and spices. In very severe cases patients have been known to actually spit-up excessive digestive acids.

The most common pathology associated with this condition is ulceration. This can be located in either the gastric mucosa or the duodenum/small intestine.

Treatment Considerations

The most effective treatment for this condition is a combination of specific spinal treatments such as would be expected from a chiropractor or osteopath and one to two tablespoons of aloe vera liquid fifteen minutes before each meal. Capsicum is also an effective healer of ulcers.

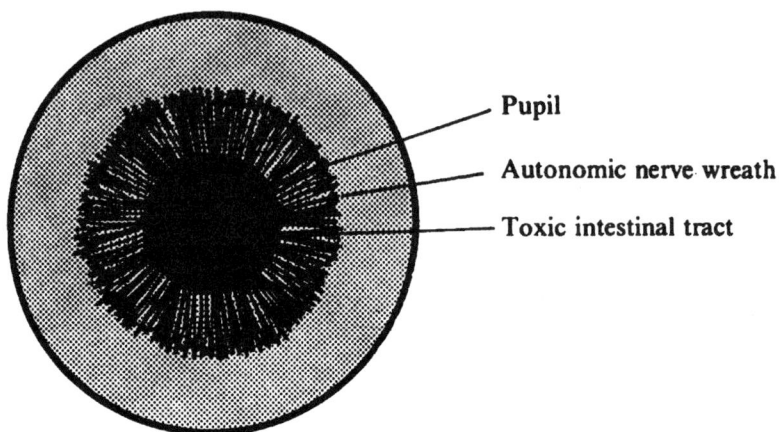

Pupil

Autonomic nerve wreath

Toxic intestinal tract

Toxic Colon

The colon easily becomes toxic because of its function in disposing of body wastes. This waste material often remains in the large intestine for months and even years, decaying more and more, producing poisons, and seeping into the body through the bowel wall. Most of this seepage is gradual except in cases where a radii solaris or radial furrow sign is present.

Most people in this country do not have a normal bowel movement or even know what a normal bowel movement is. Any person eating three "normal" sized meals per day should have a minimum of two good bowel movements per day. Anything less than this is allowing this material to remain in the body, decay and produce large amounts of poisons that will find their way into the bloodstream.

TREATMENT CONSIDERATIONS

There are excellent herbal formulas that work to rebuild the muscle strength of the intestinal wall, step up intestinal elimination, break down these pockets, and even feed the nerves associated with the parastaltic activity necessary for elimination. A good formula consists of cascara sagrada bark, barberry bark, capsicum, ginger, golden seal root, dong quai, red raspberry leaves, turkey rhubarb root, and fennel.

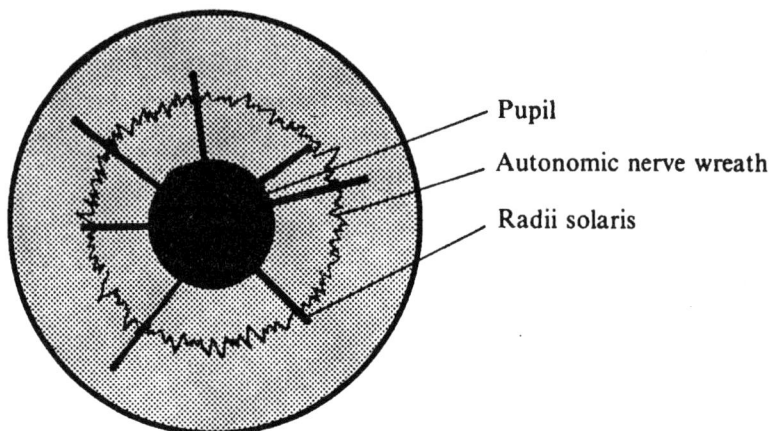

Pupil

Autonomic nerve wreath

Radii solaris

Radii Solaris

This sign is probably one of the oldest ever identified. Its use has been extremely widespread. It has been used traditionally by the many herders to maintain the health of their herds, detecting a problem prior to the manifestation of symptoms. This sign gets its name because it appears as radials from a central object—the pupil. Each of these radials indicates a low level of seepage from the intestinal tract into that area represented on the chart. Thus producing a low level of septasemia (septic blood) and inflammation.

TREATMENT CONSIDERATIONS

The bowel wall must be repaired and the musculature strengthened. The best herbal formula for this is one of Cascara Sagrada Bark, Barberry Bark, Capsicum, Ginger, Golden Seal Root, dong quai, Red Raspberry Leaves, Turkey Rhubarb Root, and Fennel.

Pupil

Autonomic nerve wreath

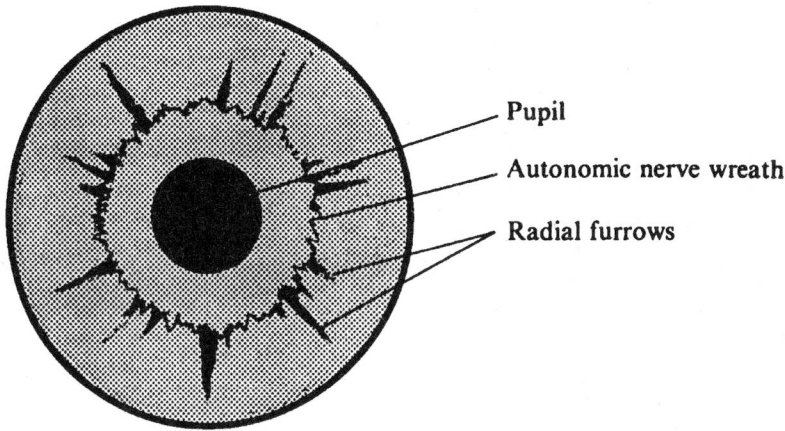

Radial furrows

Radial Furrows

Like the radii solaris, this sign indicates increased toxic material in the adjacent and surrounding tissue. However, one big difference in recognizing this condition is that, unlike the radii solaris, the radial furrow is always found outside the autonomic nerve wreath. This condition is more severe than merely a toxic colon but less severe than a radii solaris. Knowing these three different stages of toxicity of the intestinal tract enable us to evaluate the progress and stage of this condition.

TREATMENT CONSIDERATIONS

This condition responds to the same herbal combination as the radii solaris. The bowel wall must be repaired and the musculature strengthened. The best herbal formula for this is one of Cascara Sagrada Bark, Barberry Bark, Capsicum, Ginger, Golden Seal Root, dong quai, Red Raspberry Leaves, Turkey Rhubarb Root, and Fennel.

Parasites

Parasites are extremely common in this country. Anyone who has ever had a pet, a child, or both probably has at one time or another contracted parasites. These can range from pinworms to tapeworms and everything in between. People with diverticuli in their intestinal tracts and especially radii solaris and radial furrows can be expected to have quite an abundance of parasites.

TREATMENT CONSIDERATIONS

For parasitic control a marvelous formula is elecampane root, spearmint, turmeric root, ginger root, garlic bulb root, clove flower buds, wormwood and mugwort. Black walnut, herbal pumpkin and garlic should also be considered.

Before a person begins a strong parasitic purge they should first ensure that they have been having at least 2-3 very good bowel movements for at least 7-10 days. Exercise that enables the person to move up and down, such as on a home (mini-trampoline) exerciser, is excellent in assisting any eliminative problem. See chapter five for further information on parasites.

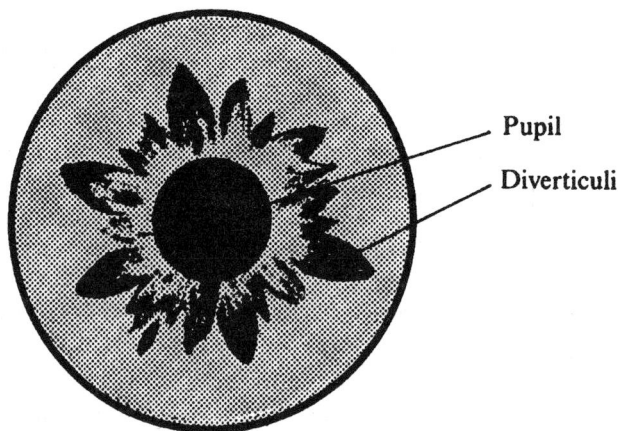

Pupil

Diverticuli

Diverticuli

Bowel pockets are formed either because of a pre-existing weakness in that area or because the large intestine is so full of waste material that the bowel was forced to balloon out. These areas become full of waste material, and become a breeding ground for harmful bacteria and parasites. Further, these areas create a constant irritation to the bowel wall in that area and are often a precursor to cancer of the colon, a form of cancer very common in this country.

Treatment Considerations

The herbal compositions suggested for the toxic colon are also very effective on this condition as well, these compositions being: Cascara Sagrada Bark, Barberry Bark, Capsicum, Ginger, Golden Seal Root, Dong quai, Red Raspberry Leaves, Turkey Rhubarb Root, and Fennel.

Autonomic Nerve Wreath

The autonomic nerve wreath (see Illustration C) is the only structure seen in the iris that is normal. All other structures, color changes, etc. are indications of an abnormal condition.

This wreath as a landmark separates what is in the intestinal tract and what is not. That way we can tell if an organ is directly involved or indirectly involved by reflexed action. Knowing this adds to our success and accuracy in analysis.

The wreath also is a direct indication of one of the most important systems of the body—the autonomic nervous system. It is this system that the brain uses to control the body. The autonomic nervous system can be thought of as an automatic system in that it controls the digesting of our food, our vision, and circulation. The list is endless.

TREATMENT CONSIDERATIONS

Those which show disturbances in the autonomic nervous system should have a complete spinal and neurological examination. The purpose of which is to locate any and all areas of nerve root pressure. They should also begin taking high levels of rice bran syrup (1 tablespoon three times a day). This syrup is extremely high in niacin and the other B-complexes. A patient deficient in niacin will tend to flush-up for a varying degree of time, depending upon the degree of their deficiency. This flushness or rash should be completely dissipated within four to six hours. As the deficiency is corrected, there will be less and less reaction to the niacin. When rice bran syrup is not available a natural source of B-complex tablets may be taken.

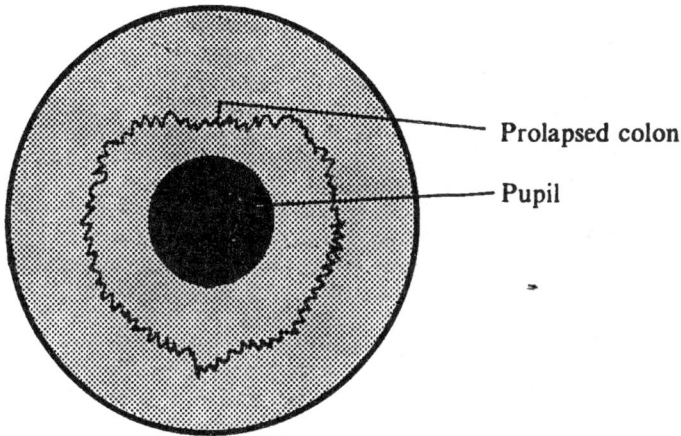

Prolapsed colon

Pupil

Prolapsed Colon

The transverse colon, because of its size and position, is often the underlying cause of many conditions, especially in those who have allowed their abdominal area to become very large. The prolapse can be detected by the flatness of the autonomic nerve wreath and by its closeness to the pupil.

TREATMENT CONSIDERATIONS

A good building formula is one consisting of Betaine HCI, pepsin, pancreatin and bile salts, as well as psyllium hulls, kelp chlorophyll, cascara sagrada bark, betonite clay, apple pectin, marshmallow root, parthenium root, charcoal, ginger root and sodium copper chlorophyllin.

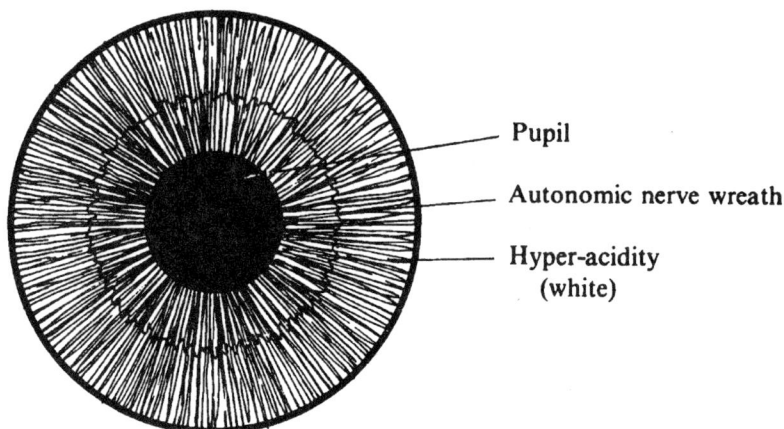

Pupil

Autonomic nerve wreath

Hyper-acidity
(white)

Hyperacidic Tissue

This is probably the most common problem found today, especially among the younger generation. There are several major causes. The end product of metabolism is CO_2 and water. Thus almost everything we eat ends up as acid in the body. Also, simple carbohydrates/sugars are extremely acid forming foods as well as meats, coffee, tea, alcohol, spices, and even citric acid fruits such as lemons, oranges, and grapefruit. One might say they thought these citric acid fruits were actually alkaline in nature. They are, but that is only when they have been completely vine-ripened. These supermarket fruits, tomatoes included, are extremely acid forming because they have not had a proper gestation period. This highly acidic condition places a very large demand upon the body to be neutralized. The body primarily uses sodium to neutralize this acidic condition. Most people in this country are extremely deficient in natural sodium. This does not mean table salt, but the sodium that is obtained from foods such as kelp, celery, parsley, etc. Because of this deficiency, the body is forced to draw upon its storehouse of this mineral. Sodium is stored primarily in two places, the stomach and the joints.

The stomach is usually the first area to give up its supply of this precious mineral, thus encouraging an "acid stomach" and the usual needs for an antacid. This may be the beginning of a gastric ulcer.

Now, as the body begins to give up more and more sodium from the joints, these joints begin to become infiltrated by calcium and become rigid, very irritated, and inflamed. Thus the real importance of the sign "high acid tissue" is that it is the underlying cause of much of the arthritis today, especially rheumatoid—the crippler.

TREATMENT CONSIDERATIONS

These people should be placed on very low acidic diets. This means to avoid the high acidic foods previously mentioned and above all, no red meat or pork. They can have all the fish or fowl they desire. They should remain off these foods completely for thirty days. After thirty days, they will normally begin feeling so good that they quickly notice the difference if they begin eating these foods again. This is usually convincing enough evidence for them to continue to avoid these products.

An excellent formula is yucca, bromelain, alfalfa, black cohosh, burdock, yarrow, capsicum, hydrangea, valerian, horsetail, white willow bark, celery seed, slippery elm bark, sarsaparilla root, and catnip.

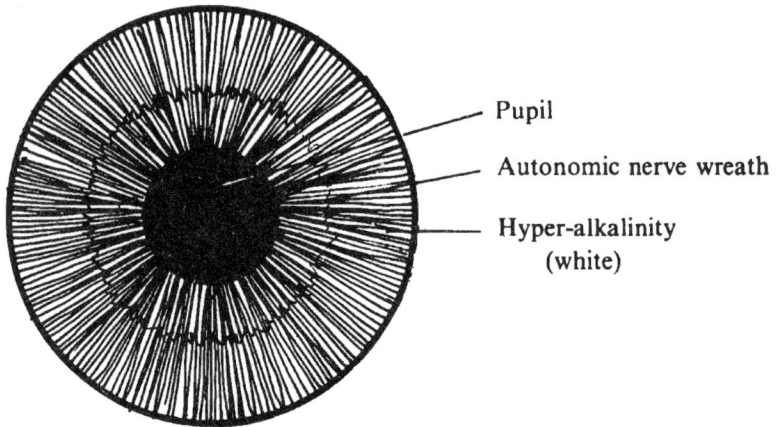

Pupil

Autonomic nerve wreath

Hyper-alkalinity
(white)

Hyperalkaline Tissues

The buildup of this alkalinity in the body cells and tissues prevents the cells from adequately disposing of waste material and likewise causes an inadequacy of taking on the desperately needed nutrition from the blood.

Hyperalkalinity is normally found in people in their 30s and up who have had a history of ulcers or an acid stomach. Most of this buildup comes from ingesting high quantities of anti-acids such as Rolaids, Tums, Alka-Seltzers, and white flour products, baking soda and similar products.

Treatment Considerations

A very good combination is juniper berries, parsley, uva ursi, marshmallow, dong quai, ginger, and golden seal root. This is also a very good formula for any kidney infection or weakness. Another very effective herbal combination is: uva ursi, parsley, dandelion, juniper berries and chamomile. Herbal potassium should also be used 2-3 times daily.

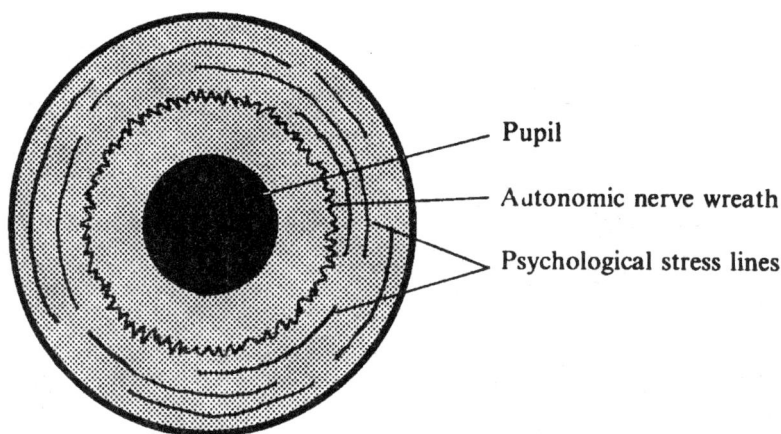

Pupil

Autonomic nerve wreath

Psychological stress lines

Psychosomatic Stress Rings

This is a very common but significant sign. These rings can be complete or partial and there can be one or more rings. They signify that a person's body is under a lot of stress. This stress can either be of psychological or physical origin.

These rings also are indicative of organs and tissue under a neurological stress, probably because they also indicate a calcium deficiency which is affecting the nerve sheath in that area. This indication of a calcium deficiency receives more comment from patients than any other sign, especially from a person who is on a high calcium diet. It is not what you take that counts, but how well your body uses what is taken.

TREATMENT CONSIDERATIONS

I find that these people respond very well to herbs and tea high in horsetail grass and alfalfa. Also a combination that contains valerian root, hops and skullcaps works well. A high B complex is necessary.

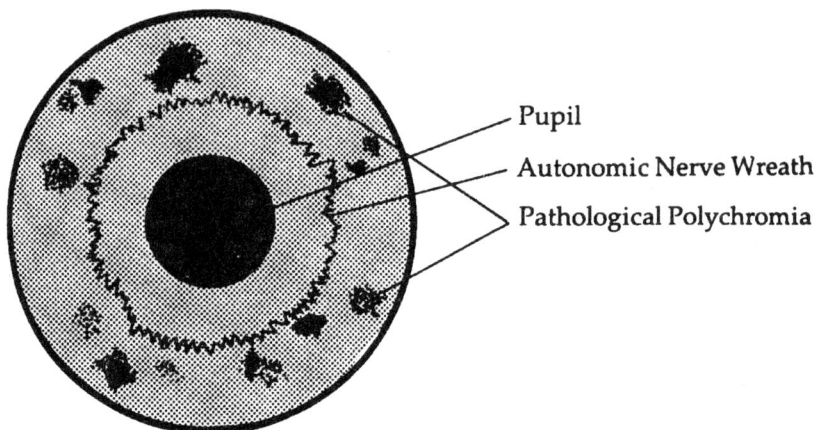

Pupil
Autonomic Nerve Wreath
Pathological Polychromia

Pathological Polychromia

In addition to the pigmentation changes of inflammation, there are certain pigmentations that appear on the iris surface at random. These had been thought in the past to be drug/mineral deposits in the tissue, but microscopic examination during cadaveral research indicates these to be deposits of various enzymes such as LDH, SGOT and others that are associated with organ cell damage. These pigmentations are termed *pathological polychromia.*

The color of these pigmentations is significant in determining which organs are involved, but the pigmentation position on the iris is not important. The emphasis should not now be on the spots, but instead, on the organ that caused them. For a complete listing of these pigmentations and their changes, refer to the companion publication of this booklet, *Practical Iridology and Sclerology,* also by Dr. Donald Bamer.

TREATMENT CONSIDERATIONS

Most of these spots will stay long after the organ which caused them has been refortified. They can usually be removed by the use of an eyewash made from the eyebright herb. The way this eyewash can be used is by emptying one capsule of the eyebright combination into a cup. Pour in 8 oz. of hot distilled water. Let it steep for eight to ten minutes, strain the mixture through a cotton cloth, let it cool, then wash out the eyes.

An exceptional herbal combination consists of cedar berries, uva ursi, licorice, mullein, capsicum, golden seal, burdock, siberian ginseng, and horseradish root. Alfalfa as a single herb is excellent to be used in conjunction with either of these combinations.

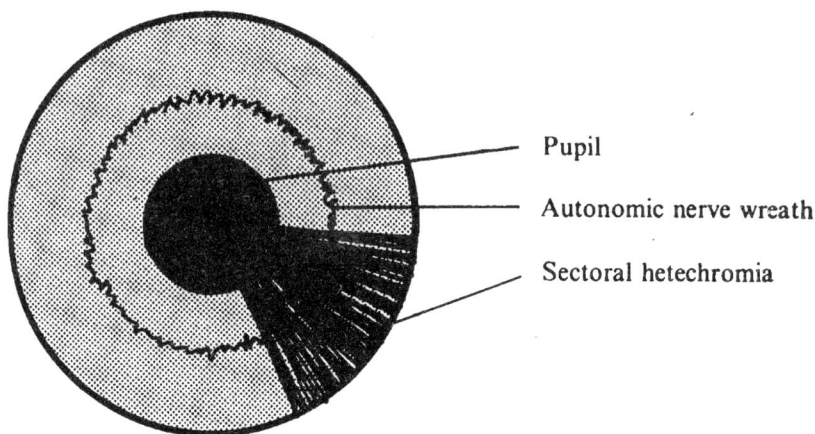

Pupil

Autonomic nerve wreath

Sectoral hetechromia

Sectoral Hetechromia

Sectoral hetechromia is the large area of a different color often seen in the eye. This can be in both eyes, but is usually predominant in only one eye. The name is very descriptive—*sectoral* (section), *hete* (different), and *chromia* (color), or a section of a different color.

Sectoral hetechromia is significant because it represents an area of the body where either a drug, heavy metal, or inorganic substance has settled. This material is a part of the tissue in that area and shows very specifically in the iris. It has often been said that this is caused by just drugs, but it can be anything chemical that the body has been unable to eliminate and thus has stored in the tissue.

TREATMENT CONSIDERATIONS

Recommended treatment for this on purified water. They should also be placed on a blood purifier combination, such as red clover, burdock, yellow dock, yarrow, dandelion, sarsaparilla or barberry.

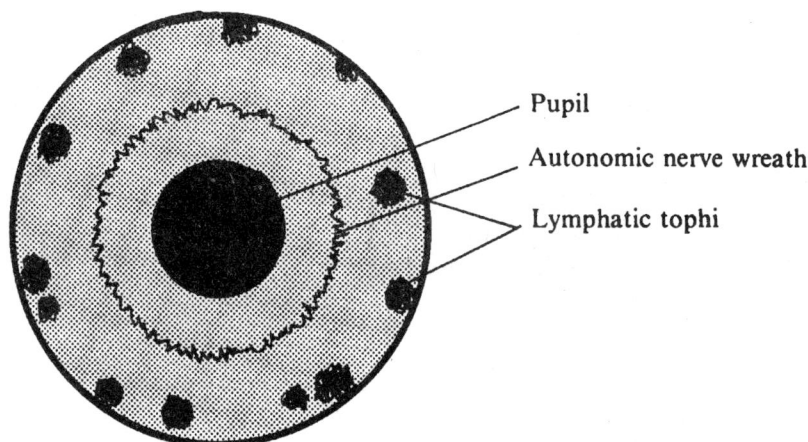

Pupil

Autonomic nerve wreath

Lymphatic tophi

Lymphatic Tophi

The lymphatic system is one of the systems of the body that man knows very little of. In fact, it was just discovered by the Russians that man actually has two hearts—the first one being to pump the blood through the system and the second being a pump for the lymphatic system. The lymphatic system is the protective system of the body as well as the system that helps the absorption of the fat soluble vitamins D, A, K, and E.

TREATMENT CONSIDERATIONS

Herbal remedies should be a combination of cascara sagrada, pau d' arco, buckthorn, red clover, peach bark, yellow dock, yarrow, sarsaparilla, barberry, dandelion, stillingia and prickly ash. Oregon grape and echinacea are also excellent blood purifiers. Rose hips as a single herb is very effective in helping the body fight infection.

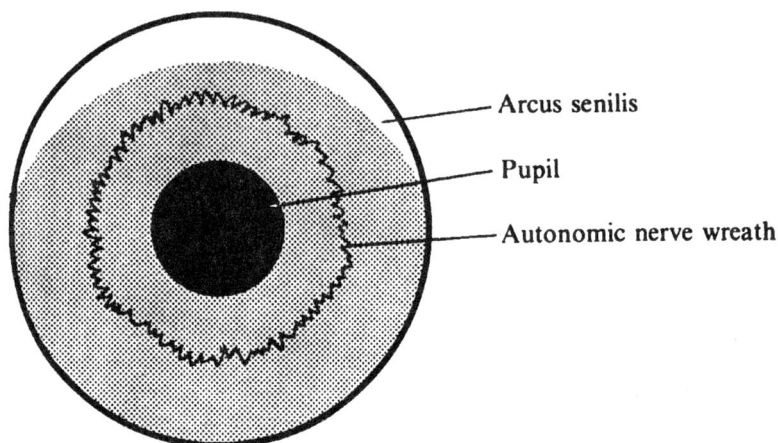

Arcus senilis
Pupil
Autonomic nerve wreath

Arcus Senilis

The arcus senilis sign was at one time only seen in those who are senile or thought to be senile. It is seen as a white hat covering approximately the upper one third of the iris. The white area is on the edge of the iris. This outer area is classed as Zone #6 and is representative of the circulatory zone. Thus it tells what is in the arteries and along the artery walls.

This sign indicates partial blockage in the arteries of the head and neck primarily. These vessels begin to plaque from triglycerides, inorganic sodium, and various other types of material that collect and create a blockage of the arteries. This sign can be seen at any age today and is indicative of a circulatory deficiency to the brain. This reduced blood flow to the brain cells is what is being found to be the cause of senility. It is a very gradual process but detectable through the use of an iris examination.

TREATMENT CONSIDERATIONS

An herbal product that nourishes and cleans the circulatory system containing vitamins, minerals, glandular extracts, amino acids and herbs should be used as an oral chelation therapy. A combination of ginkgo and gotu kola may be helpful as well. Vitamin E, 800-1000 IUs per day, will also enhance the oxygenation of the brain cells. A B-complex capsule should be taken at least 2-3 times daily. Slant board and rebounding types of exercising are a must with this condition. Exercise should be for no less than 5 minutes twice a day. Exercise again is highly recommended; three to five minutes of gentle exercise on the "Rebounder" or similar exercise unit is very beneficial. The patient should lie on a slant board twice a day for five to fifteen minutes, thus reversing the gravitational pull on the body and allowing an increased blood flow to the brain. This is also very beneficial to all that stand a great deal of the time.

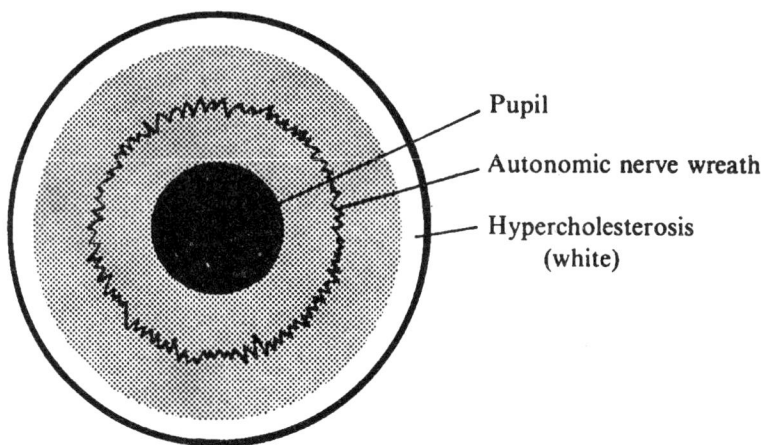

Pupil

Autonomic nerve wreath

Hypercholesterosis
(white)

Hypercholesterosis

This sign is like the arcus senilis but now extends around the complete eye. The person's vascular system is much more involved now and can create circulatory blockage anywhere in the body. In the early stages the arteries are said to be atheroscleratic, but once this condition has progressed it soon becomes one of arteriosclerosis. The extent of involvement can be estimated by the brilliance of the reflexed light from this area and the thickness of the sign.

TREATMENT CONSIDERATIONS

Like the arcus senilis, these people require more exercise and should use a nutritional herbal oral chelation product. This sign is often seen in the salt user. Salt must be removed from their diet. An organ that usually is highly involved here is the liver. An excellent combination for the liver is rose hips, red beet root, barberry, horseradish, dandelion, parsley, and fennel.

Pupil

Autonomic nerve wreath

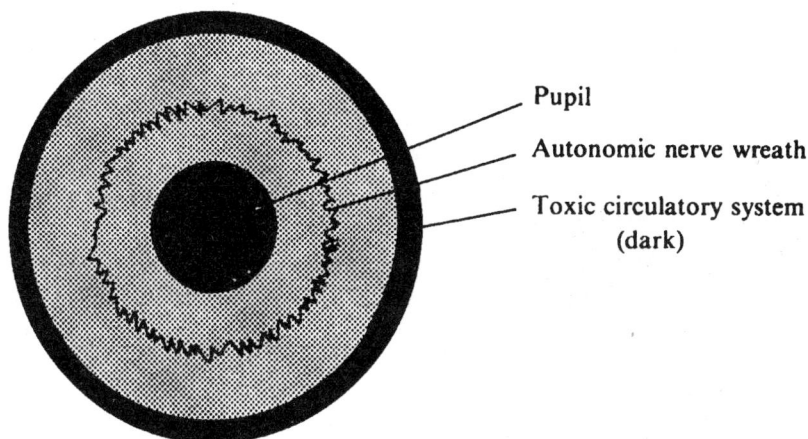

Toxic circulatory system
(dark)

Toxic Circulatory System

The circulatory system is usually involved in any case of tox-icity. It becomes more like a sewer system than a circulatory system. This is because the blood constantly (in a toxic situa-tion) has toxins seeping into it from both the large and small intestines. This material is being carried to all parts of the body. When the circulatory system is toxic, the circulatory zone will appear very dark. This is thought to be reflexing from the venous portion of the circulatory system.

TREATMENT CONSIDERATIONS

The circulatory system will begin cleansing itself very well on any one of several blood cleansers. An outstanding blood purifier is: Red Clover, Burdock, Yellow Dock, Yarrow, Dandelion, Cascara Sagrada, Barberry, Sarsaparilla, Pau d' Arco, Buckthorn, Peach Bark, Stillingia and Prickly Ash. Single herb boosts include Burdock or Echinacea.

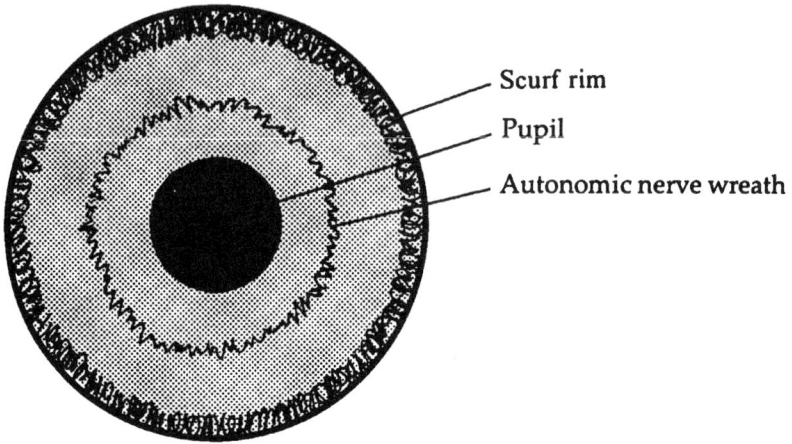

- Scurf rim
- Pupil
- Autonomic nerve wreath

Scurf Rim

The very outside of the iris is representative of the skin. Whenever the skin becomes weak or involved in being unable to shed its outer coat, the epidermis (which is dead skin), the skin becomes very congested. This congestion is reflexed into the iris as looking a bit cloudy, scurfy around the iris, thus the term scurf ring/rim.

The skin (even though not usually thought as such) is the largest organ of the body. The skin becomes very susceptible to what is occurring on the outside of it as well as the inside. On the outside it is constantly being abused by soaps and creams that clog the pores and in many cases cause much localized irritation. On the inside, the skin is a source of drainage for toxic materials that cannot escape through the normal channels. Thus many skin conditions are caused by various eliminating organs not preforming their job adequately and the skin must try to secrete the overload. This is especially true for the kidneys. If the kidneys are not eliminating its acids adequately, especially uric acid, the person will develop open, running sores on the skin that in many cases even smell like urine.

Treatment Considerations

When considering treating the skin, one must first ensure that all of the organs of elimination are functioning adequately (kidneys, lungs and alimentary tract). Also, only a very pure soap should ever be used on the skin. I prefer a soap made of Vitamins E, A, and D. The person should lather up very well with this soap each time it is used. He or she should be taking at least two showers daily, morning and evening. Prior to showering the skin should be brushed with a loofah or a dry rough washcloth. There are also some very good skin brushes which can be purchased at most health food stores.

The shower should be started with warm water then increase to hot. Stay in that temperature long enough to produce a good sweat. Lather during this period, then rinse and decrease the water temperature to cool and finish with cold. This allows the skin to go through its complete cycle of opening and closing. A person having a skin problem is usually quite deficient in the B-complexes. B-complex tablets should be taken 2-3 times daily.

Another requirement of the skin is for particular minerals and trace minerals that are usually very deficient in the American diet, these being silicon and sulfur. There are several herbal compositions that are very rich in these items. One combination for the skin includes the following herbs: dulse, horsetail, sage and rosemary. This combination of herbs feeds the skin with what the organ requires and at exactly the correct amount. Anytime the skin is being fortified, a blood purifier such as chaparral or red clover should be used in conjunction.

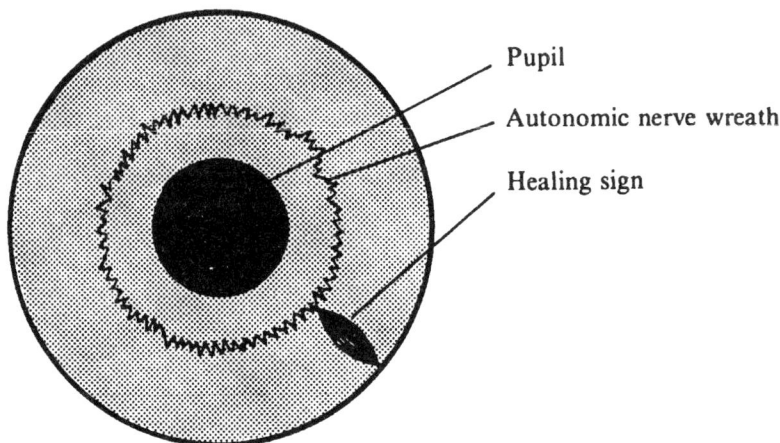

Pupil

Autonomic nerve wreath

Healing sign

Healing Crisis

When the body is actively fighting a condition there is a temperature increase, pain, and similar symptoms. We know our body is fighting something. If we will just aid our bodies by giving it rest, light nutrition, and increase our elimination, the body will handle the condition effectively.

But if we interfere and take drugs or other things that force our temperature temporarily down, this inhibits the body from ever getting rid of the original condition completely. Now we have created a chronic state in the area of the original problem. Because of its chronicity, this area will always give us problems until finally strengthened again (with our help) to the point of the increased temperature so that the body can now handle this problem completely, as it should have done in the beginning. The return to the original condition is what is termed a "healing crisis." This is what should be hoped for and worked towards with each chronic area of the body.

GLOSSARY OF TERMS

Note: These terms deal with general iridology *and* sclerology practices and techniques.

Anatomic Nerve Wreath The only structure in the iris that is normal, being a key in determining how severe other signs are in their indications of abnormal conditions.

Arcus Senilis Sign indicating senility and conditions within the arteries, like blockage in the head or neck arteries.

Colon, toxic Sign denoting toxic state in the colon, usually as a result of material remaining in intestines for long periods of time.

Cornuncle The small fatty "ball" in the corner of the eye, often the first part of the eye to show signs of disorder.

Crypt Usually seen in glandular zone, often associated with glandular disorders such as diabetes, mellitus, hypoglycemia, etc.

Defect Signs Seen as only one of the organ signs, and denotes a much more serious condition than that of a *weakness*.

Diverticuli Sign indicating pockets in the intestine full of waste material, often becoming a breeding ground for harmful bacteria and parasites.

Healing Crisis Sign indicating a crisis of healing in a particular area of the body.

Honeycomb Indicates a functional problem of metabolism occurring at that location.

Hyperalkaline Tissue Sign indicating abnormal conditions within the tissues of a particular area of the body.

Hypercholesterosis Sign similar to the arcus senilis, except extending around the complete eye. Denote's circulatory blockage in a particular area of the body.

Iridology The science that uses the iris of the eye to diagnose and monitor tissue changes that are occurring or have occurred within the body.

Leaf Lacuna Seen in the thoraic region of the eye, associated with lung or heart weakness.

Liver Stake This sign is often seen in the liver zone, shown as a triangle on the outer edge of the iris and the tip points toward the pupil.

Kidney Medussa Seen in kidney zone, indicating inherited kidney weakness.

Lymphatic Tophi Spots or freckles indicating congestion or dysfunction of the lymphatic systems.

Open Crypt Can be seen anywhere in the iris, used in conjunction with the crypt.

Open Lacuna Used in conjunction with the Leaf Lacuna, indicating an area that is weaker.

Opthalmic-Somatic Analysis Study of the whole eye, as opposed to using only the iris in diagnosing and monitoring conditions in the body.

Parasites Usually shown in the signs of radii solaris or radial furrows.

Pathological Polychromia These indicate organ cell damage, appearing as freckles or dark spots.

Pupil The opening in the eye that allows light to enter.

Pupillary Response Used to evaluate sphincter control throughout the body

Psychosomatic Stress Rings Sign indicating a particular area is under much stress, and can be of psychological or physical origin.

Radial Furrows Sign indicating increased toxic material in the adjacent and surrounding tissue, usually seen outside the autonomic nerve wreath.

Radii Solaris Indicates a low level of seepage from the intestinal tract into a particular area represented on the iridology chart.

Sclerology System of analysis using the white part of the eye to monitor and diagnose conditions within the body.

Sclera The white part of the eye, containing vessels important in diagnosis.

Scurf Rim Sign indicating congestion of the epidermis, usually by dead skin cells. Indicates weak skin condition.

Sectoral Heterochromia A large area in the eye that is a different color than the rest of the eye, usually seen in only one eye.

Somatic Constitution Pattern changes within the fibers of the iris, usually designated by three levels or categories: good, fair and poor.

Stomach, hypoactive The sign denoting dysfunction in the gastrointestinal tract, either showing overactivity or underactivity.

Stomach, hyperactive Same sign as hypoactive stomach, usually a result of ulcers, heartburn or other sensitivity problems.

Toxic Circulatory System Sign denoting seepage of toxins into the circulatory system, often affecting all areas of the body.

CASE STUDIES

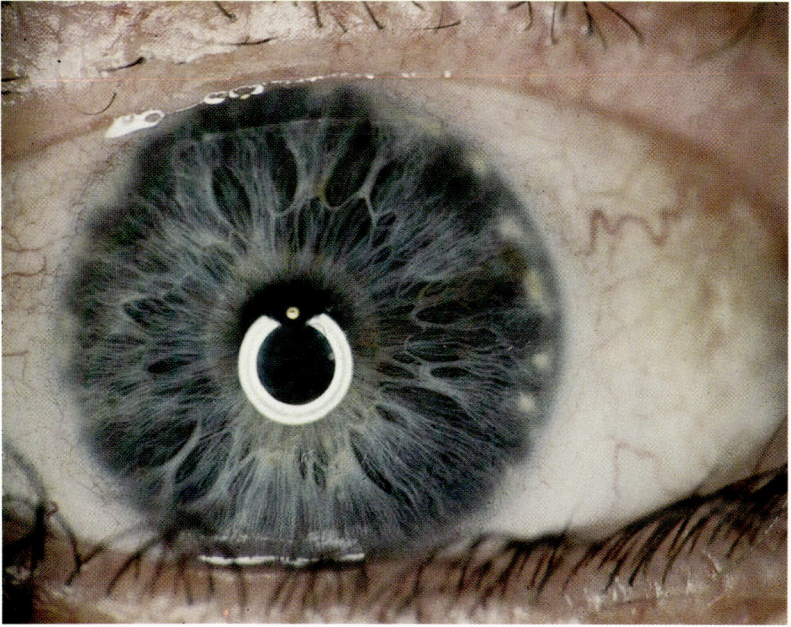

CASE STUDY 1

* Heart
* Immune System
* Brain
* Liver
* Stomach

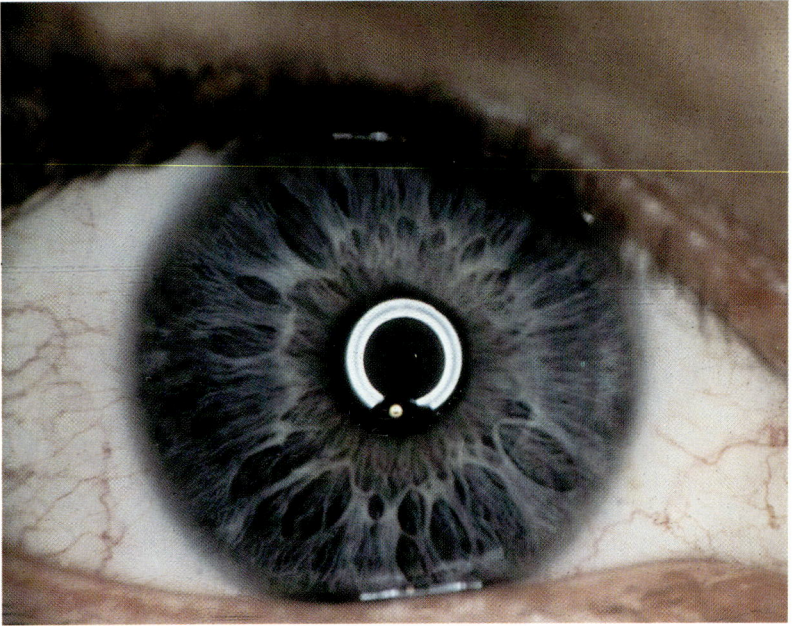

Case Study 2

* Lungs
* Liver
* Ovaries
* Arthritis
* Stomach
* Brain

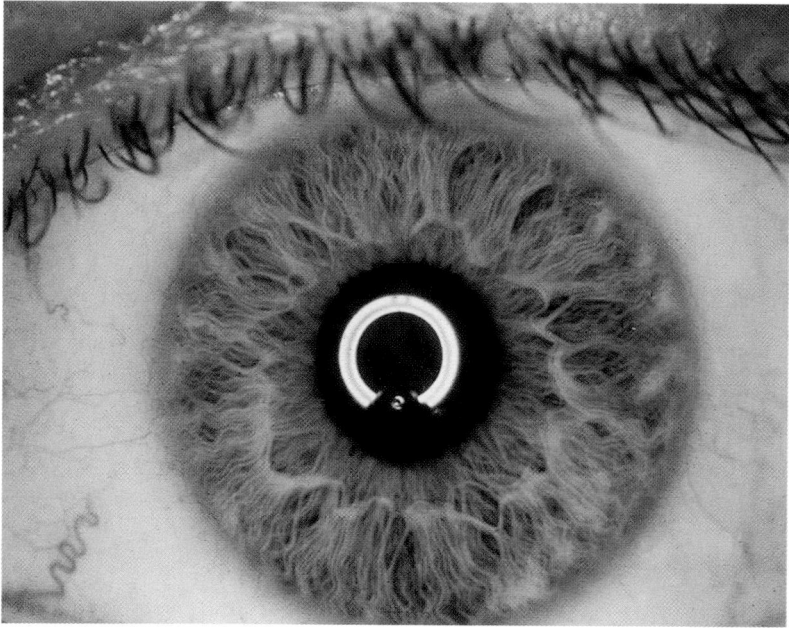

CASE STUDY 3

* Heart
* Possible Brain Tumor
* Immune Congestion
* Blood Pressure Problem

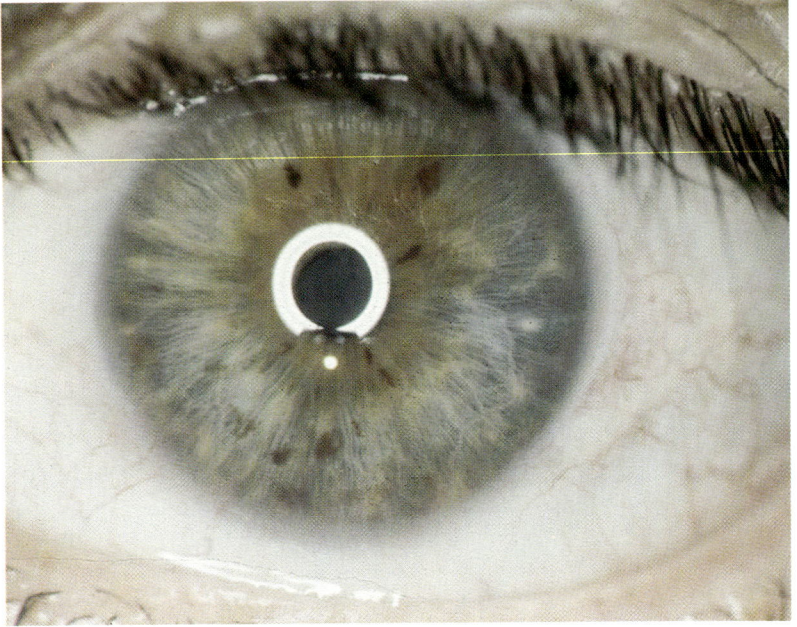

Case Study 4

* Liver
* Weak Immune System
* Arthritic
* Stomach

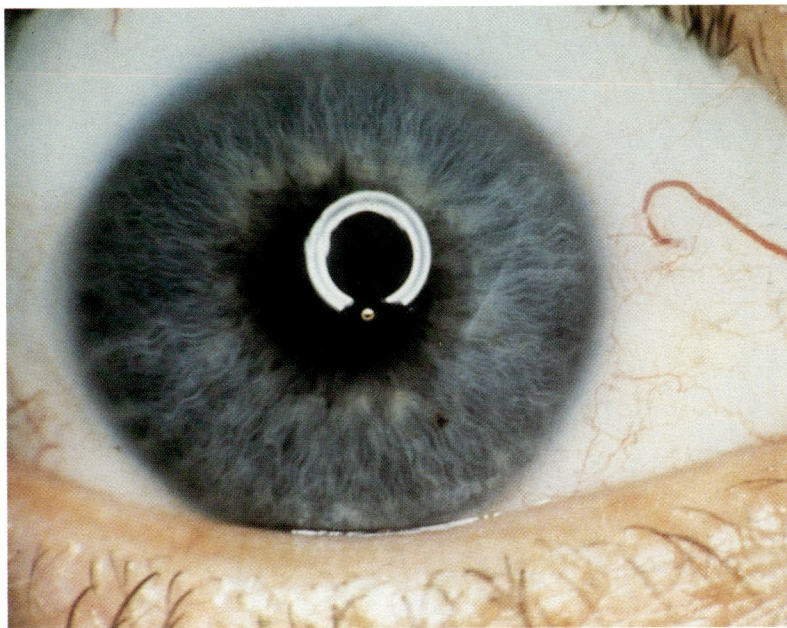

CASE STUDY 5

* Food Allergies
* Arthritic
* Poor Digestion
* Index Vessels
* Pancreas

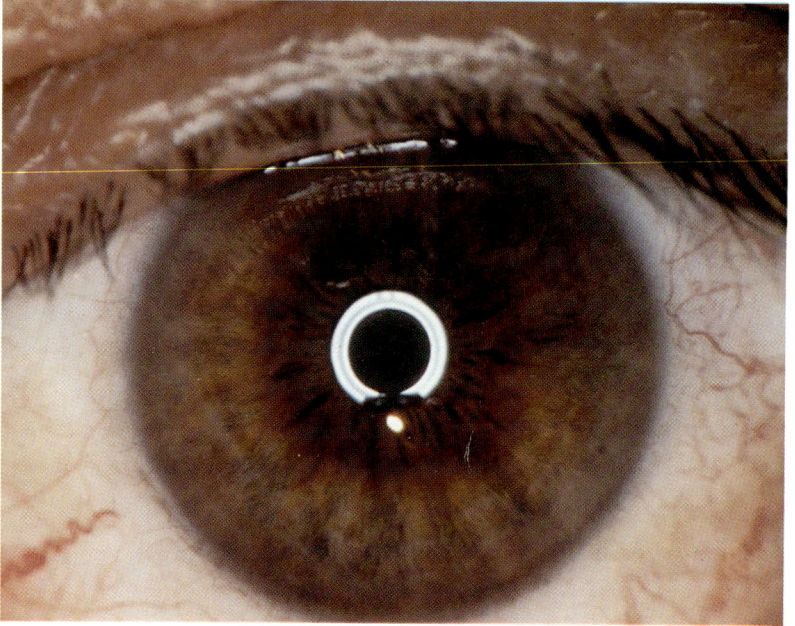

CASE STUDY 6

* Heart
* Diverticuli
* Weak Immune System
* Index Vessel
* Food Allergies

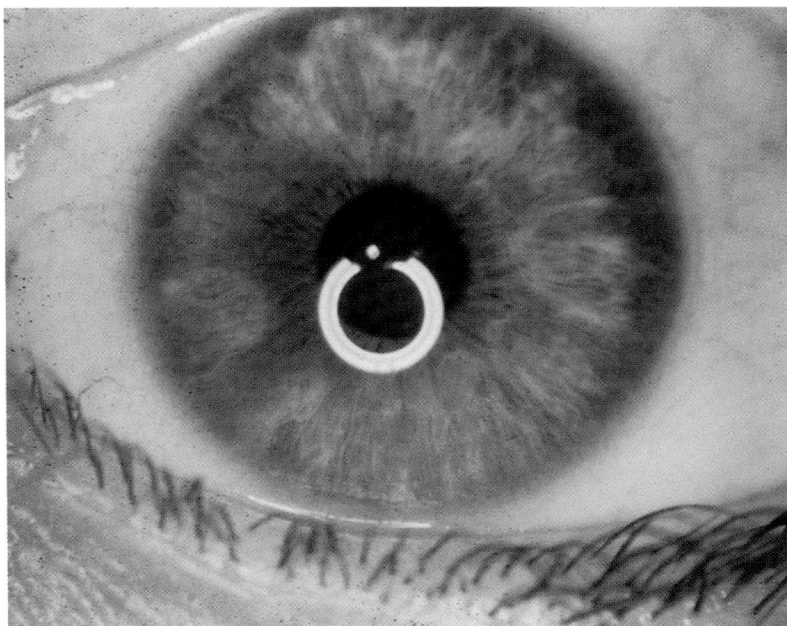

Case Study 7

* Drug Deposit
* Sectoral Hetechromia
* Arthritic
* Lymphatic (Immune) Congestion

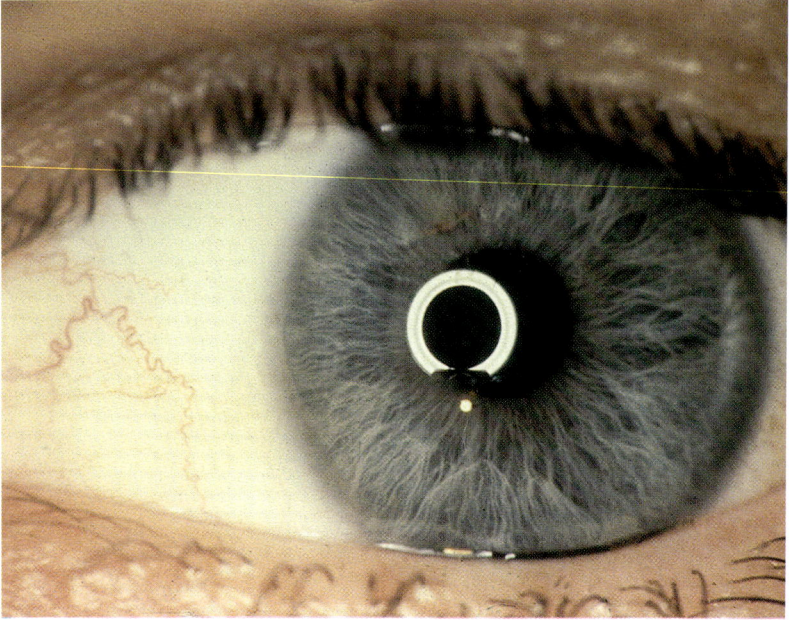

CASE STUDY 8

* Stomach
* Heart
* Lungs
* Arthritic
* Cranial Nerve Pressure

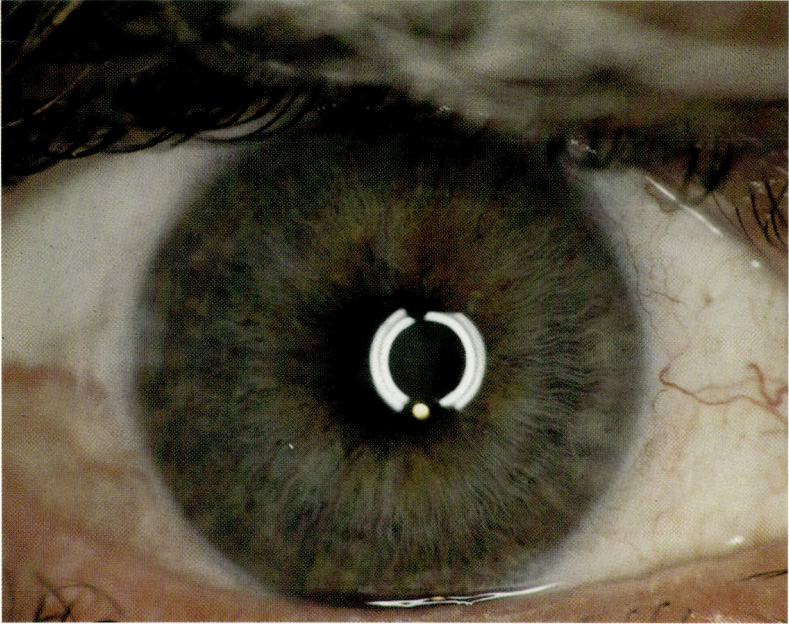

CASE STUDY 9

* Pituitary
* Ovary
* Toxic Colon
* Index Vessel
* Spiral Vessel

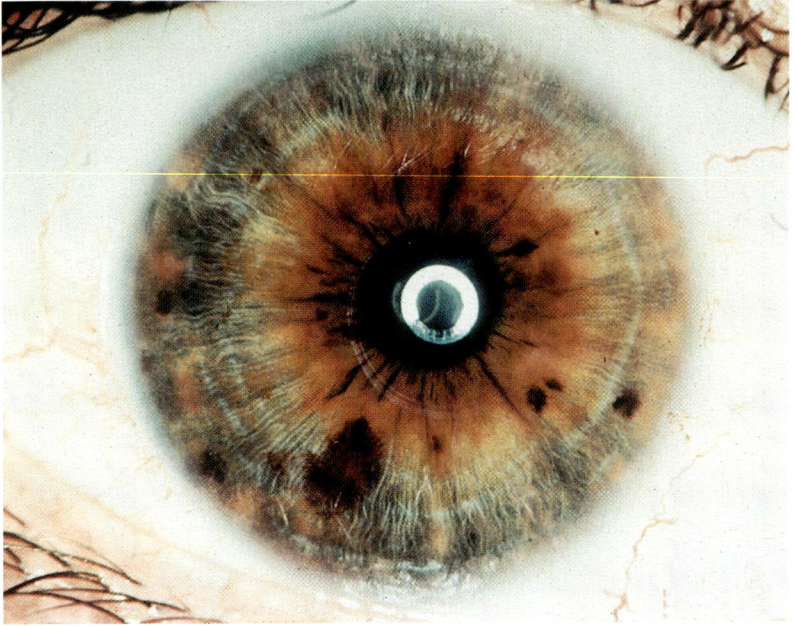

CASE STUDY 10

* Liver/Toxic Colon
* Physical/Emotional Stress
* Possible Parasites
* Possible Cancer

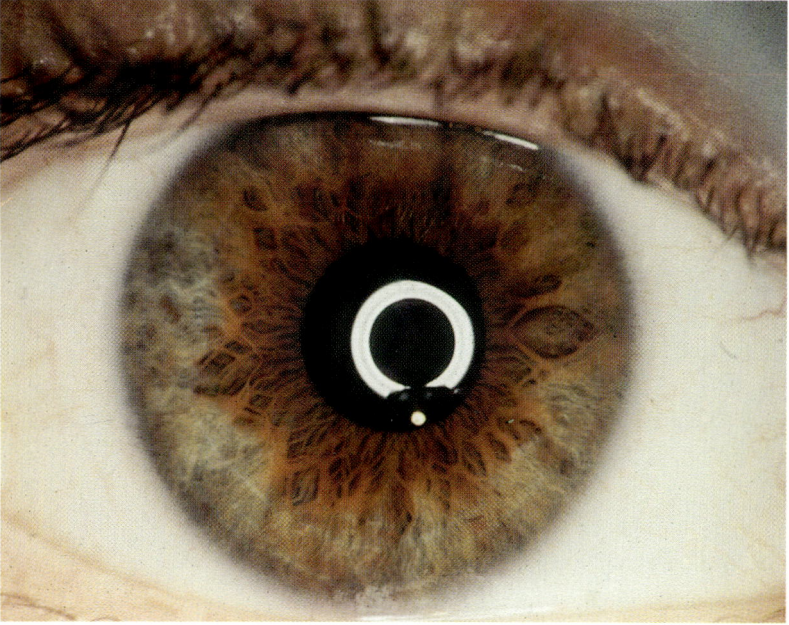

CASE STUDY 11

* Toxic Colon
* Blood Pressure
* Lung Weakness
* Liver Problem
* Brain

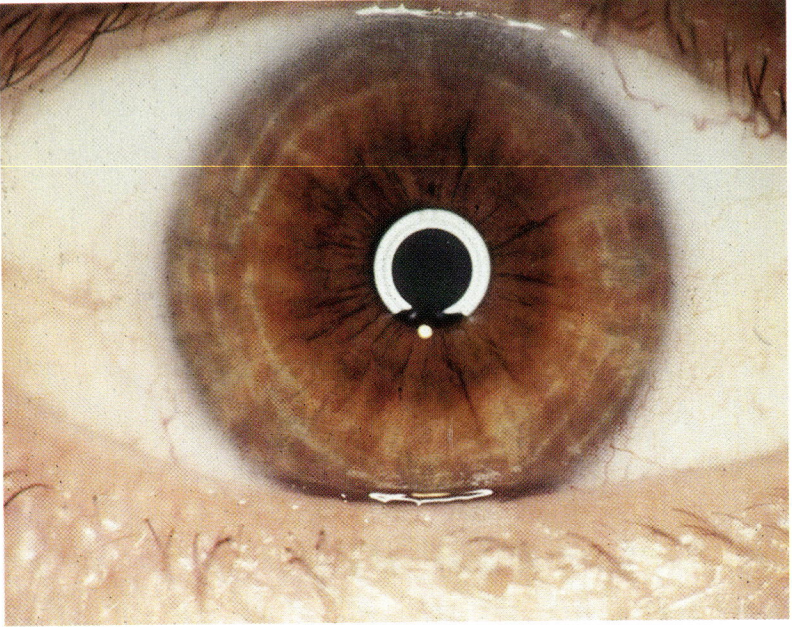

CASE STUDY 12

* Toxic Colon
* Physical/Emotional Stress
* Poor Digestion
* Adrenals

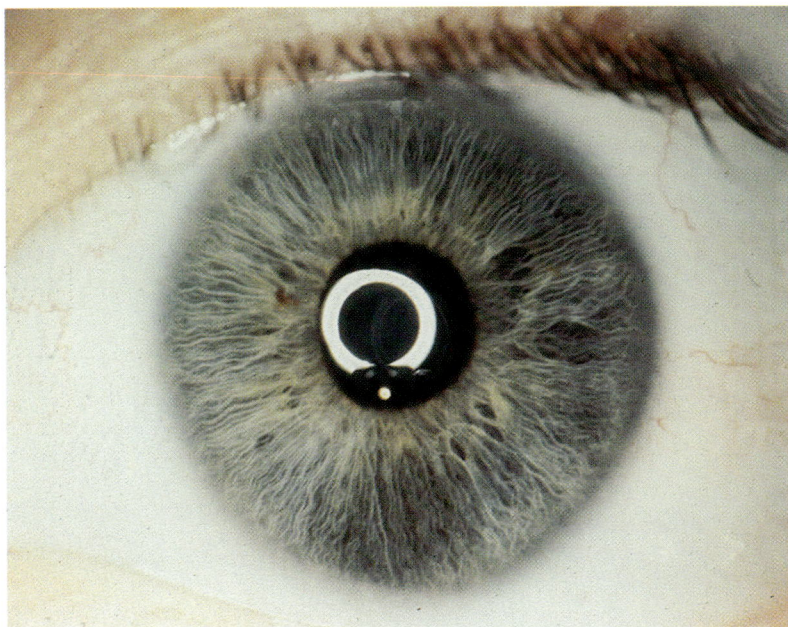

CASE STUDY 13

* Poor Brain Circulation
* Heart Weakness
* Kidney Problems
* Acidic
* Arthritic

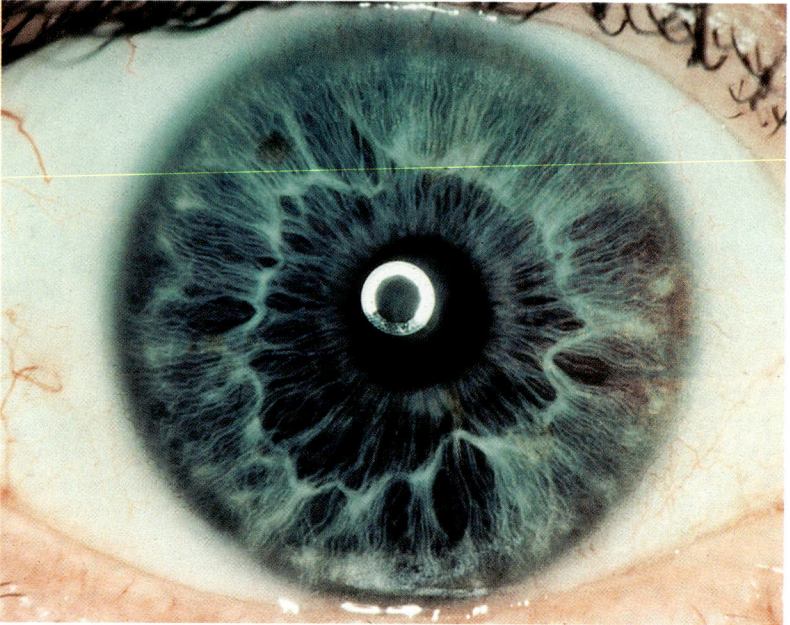

CASE STUDY 14

* Acidic Stomach
* Weak Colon
* Bowel Pockets
* Kidney Weakness

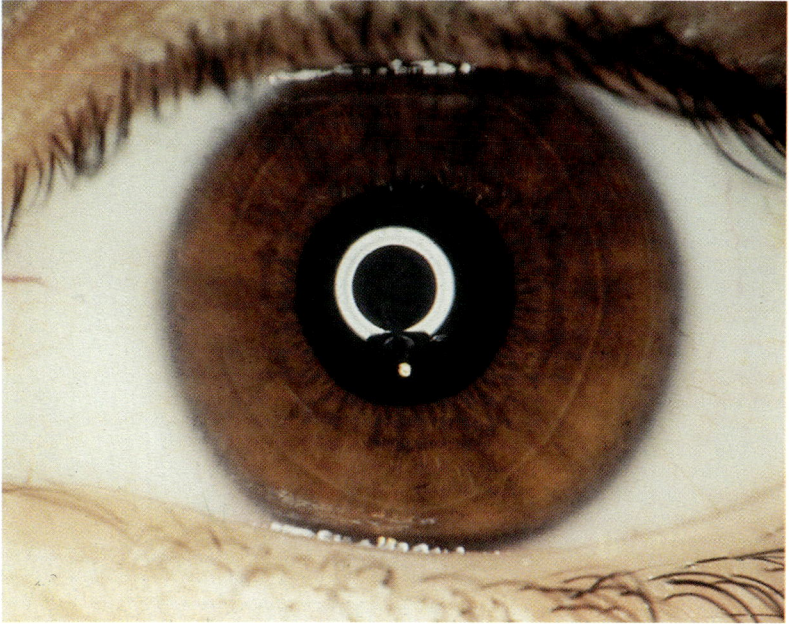

CASE STUDY 15

* Weak Adrenals
* Extreme Stress
* Toxic Colon
* Poor Digestion

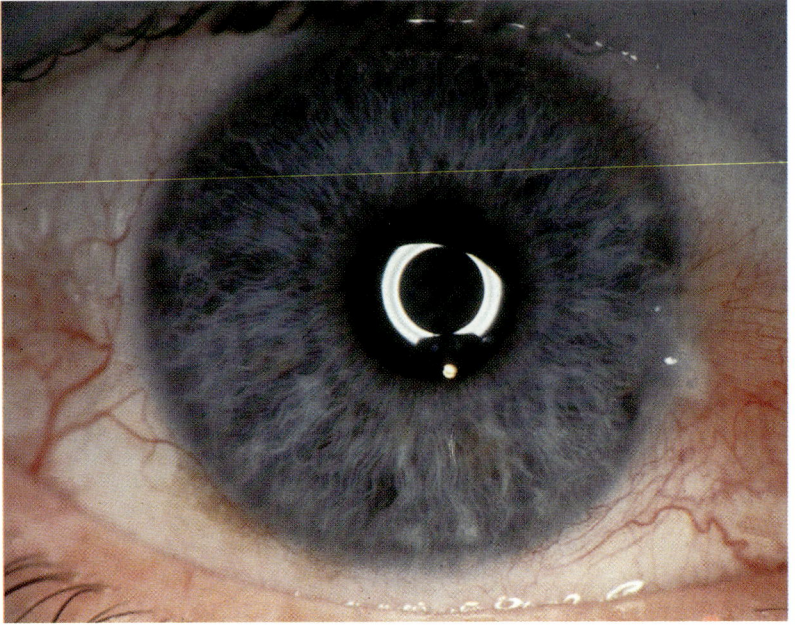

Case Study 16

* Acidic
* Arthritic
* Liver Problems
* Allergies
* Pterygium